Plant Based Meal Plan Cookbook

A Step-By-Step Guide To Quick & Easy Everyday Recipes For Busy People On A Plant Based Diet And A Plant-Based Meal Plan

Jason Canon

TABLE OF CONTENTS

Introduction

Thank you very much for purchasing this cookbook.

The diet that I am going to propose to you is healthy and balanced which guarantees weight loss without sacrificing taste, and will also make you regain the energy you didn't think you had anymore. Incorporating these foods into your diet will ensure that you can go back to doing all those activities you previously didn't think you could do anymore. Well, it's time to brush up on those hobbies and things you like to do, because on the plant base you will have more energy for your daily work and play! The mental clarity and sharpness of thought that accompany it are also positive effects you will have as a result of the diet. I really hope my recipes can help you on your weight loss journey.

Enjoy.

Breakfast Recipes

Biscuits with Mushroom Gravy

Preparation time: 45 minutes

Cooking time: 28 minutes

Servings: 16 biscuits

Ingredients:

Biscuits:

2 cups whole wheat pastry flour

2 teaspoons baking powder

2 teaspoons baking soda

3/4 teaspoon sea salt

1 cup unsweetened almond milk

1 tablespoon lemon juice

1/2 cup cashew cream (1/2 cup water blended with 1/2 cup-soaked raw cashews)

Gravy:

3 tablespoons water for sautéing vegetables

1/2 cup onion, finely chopped

1 clove garlic, minced

2 cups cremini mushrooms, chopped

2 cups low-sodium vegetable broth

1 teaspoon of sea salt

1/2 teaspoon black pepper

1/4 cup unsweetened almond milk

1/4 cup whole wheat flour

Directions:

Preheat oven to 425°F. Line a baking sheet with parchment paper. For the biscuits, mix the dry ingredients.

Mix the almond milk, lemon juice, and cashew cream in a separate bowl. Combine both dry and wet ingredients.

Form into flat circles of dough and place on the baking sheet—Bake for 7 to 8 minutes.

For the gravy, water sauté chopped onions and garlic until golden. Put the mushrooms, then cook within a few more minutes.

Put in the vegetable broth, salt, plus pepper. Add in the almond milk. Whisk in the flour and keep stirring over low heat until the gravy thickens for approximately 15 to 20 minutes.

Nutrition:

Calories 116

Fat 4g

Carbohydrate 17g

Protein 5g

Breakfast Potato Casserole

Preparation time: 15 minutes

Cooking time: 1 hour & 10 minutes

Servings: 10

Ingredients:

Sauce:

1/2 cup unsweetened almond milk

1 yellow bell pepper, chopped

1/4 cup raw cashews

1/2 cup nutritional yeast

1/2 teaspoon spicy brown mustard

1/2 teaspoon paprika

1/2 teaspoon turmeric

1 1/2 teaspoons sea salt

1/4 teaspoon black pepper

Dash of cayenne pepper

Casserole:

3 tablespoons water for sautéing vegetables

1 small yellow onion, diced

1 small red bell pepper, diced

1 small orange bell pepper, diced

7 gold potatoes, chopped into small cubes

Directions:

Preheat oven to 350°F. Set aside a 9x13 casserole dish. Place all sauce ingredients into a blender. Blend at high speed until smooth. Set aside.

Heat-up a large nonstick skillet over medium-high heat. Sauté onion until softened.   Stir in bell peppers and continue to sauté until the vegetables become tender. Add in the potatoes.

Allow mixture to heat through for a couple of minutes. Add the blended sauce mixture and stir to combine evenly.

Transfer potato and vegetable mixture to the casserole dish. Cover with foil—Bake for 45 to 50 minutes.

Uncover and continue to bake for an additional 15 to 20 minutes or until the top is golden brown. Remove from oven and serve.

Nutrition:

Calories 173

Fat 3g

Carbohydrate 30g

Protein 8g

Southwestern Tofu Scramble

Preparation time: 15 minutes

Cooking time: 10 minutes

Servings: 4

Ingredients:

14 ounces extra-firm tofu

1/4 cup low-sodium vegetable broth

1 red onion, diced

1 red bell pepper, thinly sliced

1/2 cup cremini mushrooms, chopped

1/4 cup nutritional yeast

1 teaspoon garlic powder

1 teaspoon cumin powder

1/2 teaspoon smoked paprika

1/2 teaspoon chili powder

1/2 teaspoon crushed red pepper

1/4 teaspoon turmeric

3/4 teaspoon sea salt

Black pepper to taste

Optional toppings: salsa, cilantro, hot sauce

Directions:

Pat tofu dry and absorb any excess liquid with a paper towel or clean cloth. Set aside. Heat a large skillet over medium heat.

Sauté the onions, red bell pepper, and mushrooms in the vegetable broth for approximately 5 minutes.

Take the tofu and crumble it into bite-sized pieces into the skillet. Add in the nutritional yeast and seasonings and cook for another 5 to 7 minutes until tofu is slightly browned.

Top with salsa, cilantro, or hot sauce. Serve immediately with breakfast potatoes, toast, or fruit.

Nutrition:

Calories 116

Fat 2g

Carbohydrate 11g

Protein 14g

Gorgeous Green Smoothie

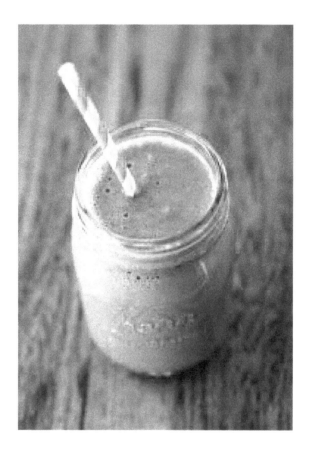

Preparation time: 5 minutes

Cooking time: 0 minutes

Servings: 2

Ingredients:

¼ cup nut or seed butter

2 frozen bananas, peeled

4 cups tightly packed shredded leafy greens

2 tablespoons chia seeds

Directions:

Combine all the fixings in a blender and add 3 cups of water. Purée for 30 seconds to 1 minute, until most of the green flecks have disappeared and the texture is smooth and creamy.

Nutrition:

Calories: 380

Fat: 22g

Protein: 12g

Carbs: 41g

Lunch Recipes

Roasted Vegetables and Tofu Salad

Preparation Time: 10 minutes

Cooking Time: 25 minutes

Servings: 4

Ingredients:

For the salad:

2 cups chopped tofu, firm, pressed, drained

2 cups cooked chickpeas

4 cups spinach

2 cups broccoli floret

2 cups chopped sweet potato, peeled

2 cups Brussel sprout, halved

4 teaspoons ground black pepper

4 teaspoons salt

4 tablespoons red chili powder

1 cup olive oil

For the dressing:

2 teaspoons salt

2 teaspoons ground black pepper

4 teaspoons dried thyme

4 tablespoons lemon juice

4 tablespoons olive oil

2 teaspoons water

½ cup hummus

Directions:

Switch on the oven, then set it to 400 degrees F and let it preheat.

Take a large baking sheet, grease it with oil, and spread broccoli florets in one-fifth of the portion, reserving few florets for later use.

Add sprouts, sweet potatoes, tofu, and chickpeas as an individual pile on the baking sheet, drizzle with oil, season with salt, black pepper, and red chili powder and then bake for 25 minutes until the tofu has turned nicely golden brown and vegetables are softened, tossing halfway.

While vegetables, grains, and tofu are being roasted, prepare the dressing and for this, take a medium jar, add all of its ingredients in it, stir until well combined, and then divide the dressing among four large mason jars.

When vegetables, grains, and tofu has been roasted, distribute evenly among four mason jars along with reserved cauliflower florets and shut with lid.

When ready to eat, shake the Mason jar until salad is coated with the dressing and then serve.

Nutrition: 477 Cal 24 g Fat 5 g Saturated Fat 52 g Carbohydrates 16 g Fiber 11 g Sugars 21 g Protein;

Farro and Lentil Salad

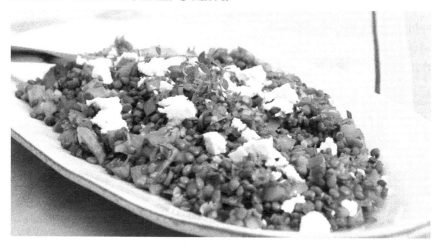

Preparation Time: 10 minutes

Cooking Time: 0 minutes

Servings: 4

Ingredients:

For the Salad:

1 cup grape tomato, halved

½ cup diced yellow bell pepper

1 cup diced cucumber,

½ cup diced red bell pepper

1 cup fresh arugula

1/3 cup chopped parsley

1 ½ cups lentils, cooked

3 ½ cups farro, cooked

For the Dressing:

½ teaspoon minced garlic

½ teaspoon salt

¼ teaspoon ground black pepper

1 teaspoon Italian seasoning

1 teaspoon Dijon mustard

2 tablespoons red wine vinegar

2 tablespoons lemon juice

1/3 cup olive oil

Directions:

Take a large bowl, place all the ingredients for the salad in it except for arugula and then toss until combined.

Prepare the dressing and for this, take a medium bowl, add all of its ingredients in it and then stir whisk until well combined.

Pour the dressing over the salad, toss until well coated, then distribute salad among four bowls and top with arugula.

Serve straight away.

Nutrition: 379 Cal 10 g Fat 2 g Saturated Fat 63.5 g Carbohydrates 11 g Fiber 2.5 g Sugars 12.5 g Protein;

Greek Zoodle Bowl

Preparation Time: 10 minutes

Cooking Time: 0 minutes

Servings: 4

Ingredients:

½ cup chopped artichokes

14 cherry tomatoes, chopped

1 medium red bell peppers, cored, chopped

4 medium zucchinis

1 medium yellow bell pepper, cored, chopped

6 tablespoons hemp hearts

1 English cucumber

6 tablespoons chopped red onion

2 tablespoons chopped parsley leaves

2 tablespoons chopped mint

For the Greek Dressing:

2 tablespoons chopped mint

1 teaspoon garlic powder

½ teaspoon salt

¼ teaspoon dried oregano

2 teaspoons Italian seasoning

3 tablespoons red wine vinegar

1 tablespoon olive oil

Directions:

Prepare zucchini and cucumber noodles and for this, spiralize them by using a spiralizer or vegetable peeler and then divide evenly among four bowls.

Top zucchini and cucumber noodles with artichokes, tomato, bell pepper, hemp hearts, onion, parsley, and mint and then set aside until required.

Prepare the dressing and for this, take a small bowl, add all the ingredients for the dressing in it and whisk until combined.

Add the prepared dressing evenly into each bowl, then toss until the vegetables are well coated with the dressing and serve.

Nutrition: 250 Cal 14 g Fat 3 g Saturated Fat 19 g Carbohydrates 5 g Fiber 9 g Sugars 13 g Protein;

Roasted Vegetables and Quinoa Bowls

Preparation Time: 10 minutes

Cooking Time: 20 minutes

Servings: 4

Ingredients:

3 cups cooked quinoa

For the Broccoli:

2 teaspoons minced garlic

4 cups broccoli florets

½ teaspoon salt

¼ teaspoon ground black pepper

4 teaspoons olive oil

For the Chickpeas:

4 teaspoons sriracha

3 cups cooked chickpeas

2 teaspoons olive oil

4 teaspoons soy sauce

For the Roasted Sweet Potatoes:

2 teaspoons curry powder

2 small sweet potatoes, peeled, ¼-inch thick sliced

1/8 teaspoon salt

2 teaspoons sriracha

2 teaspoons olive oil

For the Chili-Lime Kale:

1/2 of a lime, juiced

4 cups chopped kale

1/8 teaspoon salt

1/8 teaspoon ground black pepper

1 teaspoon red chili powder

2 teaspoons olive oil

Directions:

Switch on the oven, then set it to 400 degrees F and let it preheat.

Prepare broccoli florets and for this, take a large bowl, place all of its ingredients in it, toss until well coated, then take a baking sheet lined with parchment paper and spread florets in a one-third portion of the sheet in a row.

Add chickpeas into the bowl, add its remaining ingredients, toss until well mixed and spread them onto the baking sheet next to the broccoli florets.

Add sweet potatoes into the bowl, add its remaining ingredients, toss until well mixed and spread them onto the baking sheet next to the chickpeas.

Place the baking sheet containing vegetables and chickpeas into the oven and then bake for 20 minutes until vegetables have turned tender and chickpeas are slightly crispy, turning halfway.

Meanwhile, prepare the kale and for this, take a large skillet pan, place it over medium heat, add 1 teaspoon oil and when hot, add kale and cook for 5 minutes until tender.

Then season kale with salt, black pepper, and red chili powder, toss until mixed and continue cooking for 3 minutes, set aside until required.

Assemble the bowl and for this, distribute quinoa evenly among four bowls, top evenly with broccoli, chickpeas, sweet potatoes, and kale and then serve.

Nutrition: 415 Cal 17 g Fat 2 g Saturated Fat 54 g Carbohydrates 8 g Fiber 5 g Sugars 16 g Protein;

Dinner Recipes

Spinach and Pear Salad

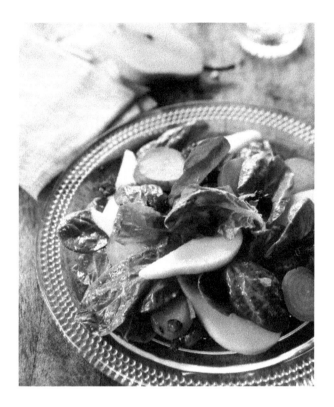

Preparation Time: 10 minutes

Cooking Time: 0 minutes

Servings: 2

Ingredients:

1 bell pepper, chopped

½ cup radishes, halved

½ cup cherry tomatoes, halved

2 cups baby spinach

2 pears, cored and cut into wedges

1 tablespoon walnuts, chopped

1 teaspoon chives, chopped

A pinch of salt and black pepper

Juice of 1 lime

Directions:

In a bowl, mix the radishes with the pepper, tomatoes and the other ingredients, toss and serve.

Nutrition: calories 143, fat 2.9, fiber 2.1, carbs 4.9, protein 3.2

Olives and Mango Mix

Preparation Time: 10 minutes

Cooking Time: 0 minutes

Servings: 2

Ingredients:

1 cup black olives, pitted and halved

1 cup kalamata olives, pitted and halved

1 cup mango, peeled and cubed

A pinch of salt and black pepper

Juice of 1 lime

1 teaspoon sweet paprika

1 teaspoon coriander, ground

1 tablespoon olive oil

Directions:

 In a bowl mix the olives with the mango and the other ingredients, toss and serve.

Nutrition: calories 68, fat 4.4, fiber 0, carbs 1.5, protein 3.3

Eggplant and Avocado Mix

Preparation Time: 10 minutes

Cooking Time: 20 minutes

Servings: 4

Ingredients:

1 pound eggplant, roughly cubed

2 avocados, peeled, pitted and cubed

1 red onion, chopped

1 teaspoon curry powder

Juice of 1 lime

½ cup crushed tomatoes

1 tablespoon olive oil

1 teaspoon salt

1 teaspoon chili powder

Directions:

 Heat up a pan with the oil over medium heat, add the onion and cook for 5 minutes.

37

Add the eggplants, avocados and the other ingredients, toss and cook for 15 minutes more.

Divide between plates and serve.

Nutrition:

calories 231

fat 7.6

fiber 8.5

carbs 9.2

protein 5.4

Red Onion, Avocado and Radishes Mix

Preparation Time: 15 minutes

Cooking Time: 12 minutes

Servings: 2

Ingredients:

2 red onions, peeled and sliced

2 avocados, peeled, pitted and sliced

1 cup radishes, halved

1 teaspoon oregano, dried

1 teaspoon basil, dried

1 tablespoon olive oil

1 teaspoon lemon juice

¼ teaspoon salt

Directions:

Heat up a pan with the oil over medium heat, add the onions, oregano and basil and cook for 5 minutes.

Add the rest of the ingredients, toss, cook for 7 minutes more, divide into bowls and serve.

Nutrition:

calories 145

fat 7.1

fiber 2.4

carbs 10.3

protein 6.2

Vegetables Recipes

Minutes Vegetarian Pasta

Preparation Time: 5 minutes

Cooking Time: 16 minutes

Servings: 4

Ingredients:

3 shallots, chopped

¼ teaspoon red pepper flakes

¼ cup vegan parmesan cheese

2 tablespoons olive oil

2 garlic cloves, minced

8-ounces spinach leaves

8-ounces linguine pasta

1 pinch salt

1 pinch black pepper

Directions:

Boil salted water in a large pot and add pasta.

Cook for about 6 minutes and drain the pasta in a colander.

Heat olive oil over medium heat in a large skillet and add the shallots.

Cook for about 5 minutes until soft and caramelized and stir in the spinach, garlic, red pepper flakes, salt and black pepper.

Cook for about 5 minutes and add pasta and 2 spoons of pasta water.

Stir in the parmesan cheese and dish out in a bowl to serve.

Nutrition:

Calories: 25;

Fat: 2.0g;

Protein: 5.2g;

Carbohydrates: 5.3g;

Fiber: 4g;

Sodium: 18mg

Asian Veggie Noodles

Preparation Time: 10 minutes

Cooking Time: 20 minutes

Servings: 4

Ingredients:

½ cup peas

1 teaspoon rice vinegar

3 carrots, chopped

1 small packet vermicelli

3 tablespoons sesame oil

1 red pepper, chopped in small cubes

1 can baby corn

1 clove garlic, chopped

2 tablespoons soy sauce

1 teaspoon ginger powder

½ teaspoon curry powder

Salt and black pepper, to taste

Directions:

Take a bowl and add ginger powder, vinegar, soy sauce, curry powder, and a pinch of salt to it.

Cook the noodles according to the instructions and drain them.

Heat the sesame oil and cook vegetables in it for 10 minutes on medium heat.

Add noodles to it and cook for 3 more minutes.

Remove from heat and serve to enjoy.

Nutrition:

Calories: 25;

Fat: 2.0g;

Protein: 5.2g;

Carbohydrates: 5.3g;

Fiber: 4g;

Sodium: 18mg

Cauliflower Latke

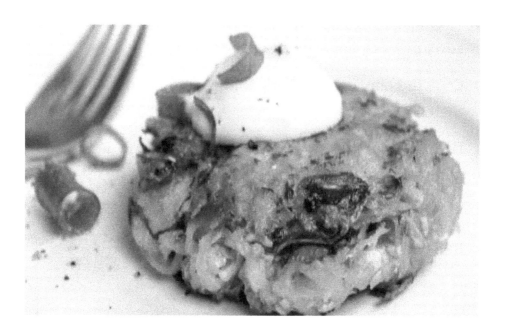

Preparation Time: 15 minutes

Cooking Time: 30 minutes

Servings: 4

Ingredients:

12 oz. cauliflower rice, cooked

1 egg, beaten

1/3 cup cornstarch

Salt and pepper to taste

¼ cup vegetable oil, divided

Chopped onion chives

Direction

Squeeze excess water from the cauliflower rice using paper towels.

Place the cauliflower rice in a bowl.

Stir in the egg and cornstarch.

Season with salt and pepper.

Fill 2 tablespoons of oil into a pan over medium heat.

Add 2 to 3 tablespoons of the cauliflower mixture into the pan.

Cook for 3 minutes each side.

Repeat until you've used up the rest of the batter.

Garnish with chopped chives.

Nutrition: 209 Calories, 1.9g Fiber , 3.4g Protein

Roasted Brussels Sprouts

Preparation Time: 30 minutes

Cooking Time: 20 minutes

Servings: 4

Ingredients:

1 lb. Brussels sprouts, sliced in half

1 shallot, chopped

1 tablespoon olive oil

Salt and pepper to taste

2 teaspoons balsamic vinegar

¼ cup pomegranate seeds

¼ cup goat cheese, crumbled

Direction:

Preheat your oven to 400 degrees F.

Coat the Brussels sprouts with oil.

Sprinkle with salt and pepper.

Transfer to a baking pan.

Roast in the oven for 20 minutes.

Drizzle with the vinegar.

Sprinkle with the seeds and cheese before serving.

Nutrition:

117 Calories

4.8g Fiber

5.8g Protein

Finger Food

Fall Fruit with Creamy Dressing

Preparation time: 25 Minutes

Cooking Time: 0 Minutes

Serving: 4

Ingredients:

Salad

Pumpkin, raw, shredded, one half cup

Pomegranate seeds, one half cup

Grapes, one cup

Apples, three, cored and cubed

Creamy Dressing

Cinnamon, one teaspoon

Lemon juice, one tablespoon

Almond yogurt, one half cup

Directions:

Mix together all of the listed Ingredients: for the dressing.

In a large-sized bowl, toss the dressing with the shredded raw pumpkin, pomegranate seeds, apples, and the dressing. Serve immediately.

Nutrition:

Calories: 161

Protein: 3g

Fat: 1g

Carbs: 40g

Summertime Fruit Salad

Preparation time: 15 Minutes

Cooking Time: 0 Minutes

Serving: 6

Ingredients:

Balsamic vinegar, two teaspoons

Lemon juice, two tablespoons

Mint, fresh chopped, one tablespoon

Blueberries, one cup

Peaches, fresh, three, peeled and sliced thin

Strawberries, one pound, cleaned and sliced thin

Directions:

Mix together in a medium-sized serving bowl the basil, blueberries, peaches, and strawberries. In a small-sized bowl, mix together the balsamic vinegar and the lemon juice.

Pour the liquid dressing over the mixed fruit and toss gently to coat all of the pieces of fruit with the dressing.

Serve immediately or keep the salad covered in the refrigerator for no longer than two days.

Nutrition:

Calories: 91

Protein: 1g

Fat: 6g

Carbs: 22g

Cherry Berry Salad

Preparation time: 10 Minutes

Cooking Time: 0 Minutes

Serving: 6

Ingredients:

Lemon juice, three tablespoons

Cardamom, one quarter teaspoon

Cinnamon, one half teaspoon

Mint, fresh, three tablespoons

Blackberries, one cup

Blueberries, one cup

Raspberries, one cup

Cherries, seeded, cut in half, one cup

Strawberries, cleaned, two cups quartered

Directions:

In a small-sized bowl, mix the spices and the lemon juice together well. In a medium-sized bowl, mix the fruits together with the lemon juice and mint mixture.

Toss the fruits gently but thoroughly to coat all of the pieces. This will store well in the refrigerator for two to three days.

Nutrition:

Calories: 113

Protein: 1g

Fat: 1g

Carbs: 27g

Fruit Salad with Sweet Lime Dressing

Preparation time: 15 Minutes

Cooking Time: 0 Minutes

Serving: 9

Ingredients:

Salad

Mint, fresh chopped, one cup

Lime juice, two tablespoons

Kiwi, five, peeled and sliced

Mangoes, two, peeled and chopped

Green grapes, one cup cut in half

Blackberries, one cup

Blueberries, one cup

Strawberries, one cup sliced

Sweet Lime Dressing

Powdered sugar, two tablespoons

Lime juice, two tablespoons

Directions:

Mix together until smooth in a small-sized bowl the powdered sugar and the lime juice.

Mix together in a large-sized bowl the fruits, then pour on the dressing and gently toss all of the fruits together well to coat all of the pieces.

This will stay good in the refrigerator for no more than one day.

Nutrition:

Calories: 50

Protein: 1g

Fat: 1g

Carbs: 12g

Asian Fruit Salad

Preparation time: 30 Minutes

Cooking Time: 0 Minutes

Serving: 8

Ingredients:

Passion fruit, one-half cup (about six of the fruit)

Papaya, one chopped

Pineapple, one cup chunked

Oranges, two separated into segments

Star fruit, three sliced thin

Mangoes, two larges, peeled and chunked

Mint, fresh, one-third cup chopped coarse

Lime juice, one third cup

Lime zest, one tablespoon

Ginger, ground, one tablespoon

Vanilla extract, one tablespoon

Brown sugar, one half cup

Water, four cups

Directions:

Mix the water and the sugar together in a medium-sized saucepan and put it over a medium to high heat until the sugar is dissolved.

Let this simmer for five minutes over a very low heat, so the sugar does not burn. Add in the vanilla extract and the ginger and stir well.

Let this cook for ten more minutes. Let the mix cool off the heat until it is room temperature, and then add in the mint, juice, and zest.

During the time the sauce is cooling mix together the remainder of the Ingredients in a large-sized bowl.

Pour the syrup mixture over the fruit in the bowl and mix gently to coat all pieces with the sauce.

Put the bowl in the refrigerator until the fruit is cold then serve.

Nutrition:

Calories: 220

Protein: 3g

Fat: 1g

Carbs: 56g

Mimosa Salad

Preparation time: 10 Minutes

Cooking Time: 0 Minutes

Serving: 8

Ingredients:

Mint, fresh, one half cup

Orange juice, one half cup

Pineapple, one cup cut into small pieces

Strawberries, one cup cut into quarters

Blueberries, one cup

Blackberries, one cup

Kiwi, three peeled and sliced

Directions:

In a large-sized bowl, mix all of the fruits together and then top with the orange juice and the fresh mint.

Toss gently together all of the fruit until they are well mixed.

Nutrition: Calories: 215 , Protein: 3g , Fat: 1g , Carbs: 49g

Honey Lime Quinoa Fruit Salad

Preparation time: 20 Minutes

Cooking Time: 0 Minutes

Serving: 6

Ingredients:

Basil, chopped, one tablespoon

Lime juice, two tablespoons

Mango, diced, one cup

Blueberries, one cup

Blackberries, one cup

Strawberries, sliced, one- and one-half cup

Quinoa, cooked, one cup

Directions:

In a large-sized bowl, mix the fruits with the cooked quinoa and mix well.

Drizzle on the lime juice and add the chopped basil and mix the fruit gently but thoroughly to coat all of the pieces.

Nutrition:

Calories: 246

Protein: 7g

Fat: 1g

Carbs: 44g

Tofu Salad Sandwiches

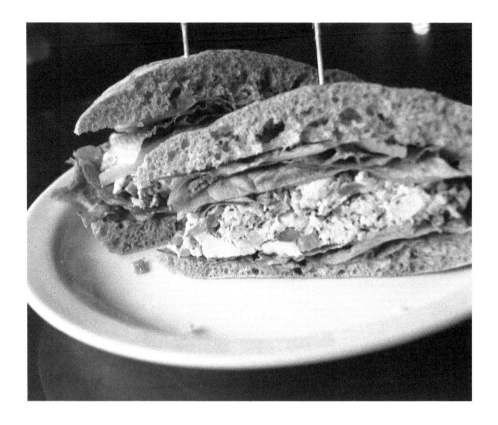

Preparation time: 15 minutes

Cooking time: 0 minutes

Servings: 6

Ingredients:

1 (14-ounce) package extra-firm tofu, drained and pressed (see here)

2 celery stalks, finely chopped

1 scallion, finely chopped

1/3 cup Cashew Mayonnaise, or store-bought nondairy mayonnaise

1 teaspoon yellow mustard

1 teaspoon freshly squeezed lemon juice

1 teaspoon ground turmeric

Salt

Freshly ground black pepper

12 slices bread of choice

1 large tomato, sliced

6 large romaine lettuce leaves

Directions:

Crumble the tofu into a medium bowl. Using a fork, gently mash it into small pieces.

Stir in the celery and scallion. Gently fold in the mayonnaise, mustard, lemon juice, and turmeric. Taste and season with salt and pepper.

Spoon the tofu mixture onto 6 slices of bread. Add the tomato slices and lettuce leaves and top with the remaining bread slices.

First-Timer tip: You can mix up your tofu salad by freezing the tofu beforehand, which makes it firmer and chewier. It also makes it a little spongy, which helps absorb dressings and sauces better. Just pop the package of tofu into the freezer. Once it's fully frozen, defrost it totally, then drain and press out the water as you normally would.

Nutrition: Calories: 247; Fat: 9g; Carbohydrates: 30g; Fiber: 5g; Protein: 13g; Sodium: 382mg;

Chickpea Salad Sandwiches

Preparation time: 15 minutes

Cooking time: 0 minutes

Servings: 4

Ingredients:

1 (15-ounce) can chickpeas, drained and rinsed, or 1½ cups cooked chickpeas (see here)

2 celery stalks, chopped

1 small carrot, grated or shredded

1/4 cup finely chopped red onion

1/4 cup finely chopped dill pickle, or pickle relish

1/4 cup Cashew Mayonnaise, or store-bought nondairy mayonnaise

1 teaspoon dried dill

½ teaspoon garlic powder

½ teaspoon onion powder

Salt

Freshly ground black pepper

8 slices bread of choice

1 large tomato, sliced

4 large romaine lettuce leaves

Directions:

Place the chickpeas in a large bowl and, using a potato masher or large fork, lightly mash them.

Gently stir in the celery, carrot, red onion, and dill pickle to combine everything.

Gently fold in the mayonnaise, dill, garlic powder, and onion powder. Taste and season with salt and pepper.

Spoon the chickpea mixture onto 4 slices of bread. Add the tomato slices and lettuce leaves and top with the remaining bread slices.

Variation tip: This recipe is reminiscent of chicken salad, but you can easily turn it into a vegan "tuna" salad by omitting the dill, garlic powder, and onion powder, and using 2 teaspoons seaweed flakes instead. You can usually find seaweed flakes in the Asian food aisle of the grocery store.

Nutrition: Calories: 320; Fat: 9g; Carbohydrates: 49g;

Fiber: 10g; Protein: 14g; Sodium: 510mg;

Soup and Stew

Sweet Potato, Corn and Jalapeno Bisque

Preparation Time: 10 minutes

Cooking Time: 15 minutes

Servings: 4

Ingredients:

4 ears corn

1 seeded and chopped jalapeno

4 cups vegetable broth

1 tablespoon olive oil

3 peeled and cubed sweet potatoes

1 chopped onion

½ tablespoon salt

¼ teaspoon black pepper

1 minced garlic clove

Directions:

In a pan, heat the oil over medium flame and sauté onion and garlic in it and cook for around 3 minutes. Put broth and sweet potatoes in it and bring it to boil. Reduce the flame and cook it for an additional 10 minutes.

Remove it from the stove and blend it with a blender. Again, put it on the stove and add corn, jalapeno, salt, and black pepper and serve it.

Nutrition:

Carbohydrates 31g

protein 6g

fats 4g

sugar 11g.

Creamy Pea Soup with Olive Pesto

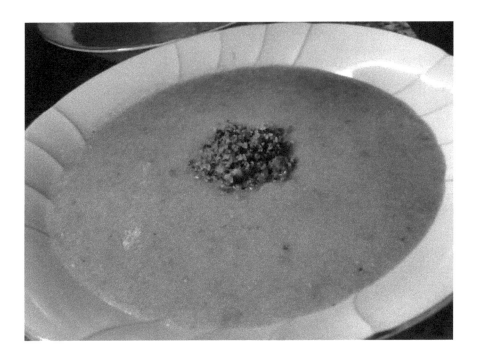

Preparation Time: 20 minutes

Cooking Time: 20 minutes

Servings: 4

Ingredients:

1 grated carrot

1 rinsed chopped leek

1 minced garlic clove

2 tablespoons olive oil

1 stem fresh thyme leaves

15 ounces rinsed and drained peas

½ tablespoon salt

¼ teaspoon ground black pepper

2 ½ cups vegetable broth

¼ cup parsley leaves

1 ¼ cups pitted green olives

1 teaspoon drained capers

1 garlic clove

Directions:

Take a pan with oil and put it over medium flame and whisk garlic, leek, thyme, and carrot in it. Cook it for around 4 minutes.

Add broth, peas, salt, and pepper and increase the heat. When it starts boiling, lower down the heat and cook it with a lid on for around 15 minutes and remove from heat and blend it.

For making pesto whisk parsley, olives, capers, and garlic and blend it in a way that it has little chunks. Top the soup with the scoop of olive pesto.

Nutrition:

Carbohydrates 23g

protein 6g

fats 15g

sugar 4g

calories 230.

Spinach Soup with Dill and Basil

Preparation Time: 10 minutes

Cooking Time: 25 minutes

Servings: 8

Ingredients:

1 pound peeled and diced potatoes

1 tablespoon minced garlic

1 teaspoon dry mustard

6 cups vegetable broth

20 ounces chopped frozen spinach

2 cups chopped onion

1 ½ tablespoons salt

½ cup minced dill

1 cup basil

½ teaspoon ground black pepper

Directions:

Whisk onion, garlic, potatoes, broth, mustard, and salt in a pan and cook it over medium flame. When it starts boiling, low down the heat and cover it with the lid and cook for 20 minutes.

Add the remaining ingredients in it and blend it and cook it for few more minutes and serve it.

Nutrition:

Carbohydrates 12g

protein 13g

fats 1g

calories 165.

Appetizer

Avocado and Tempeh Bacon Wraps

Preparation time: 10 minutes

Cooking time: 8 minutes

Servings: 4

Ingredients:

2 tablespoons extra-virgin olive oil

8 ounces tempeh bacon, homemade or store-bought

4 (10-inch) soft flour tortillas or lavash flat bread

¼ cup vegan mayonnaise, homemade or store-bought

4 large lettuce leaves

2 ripe Hass avocados, pitted, peeled, and cut into ¼-inch slices

1 large ripe tomato, cut into ¼-inch slices

Directions:

Heat-up the oil in a large skillet over medium heat. Add the tempeh bacon and cook until browned on both sides, about 8 minutes. Remove from the heat and set aside.

Place 1 tortilla on a work surface. Spread with some of the mayonnaise and one-fourth of the lettuce and tomatoes.

Thinly slice the avocado and place the slices on top of the tomato. Add the reserved tempeh bacon and roll up tightly. Repeat with remaining Ingredients and serve.

Nutrition:

Calories: 315

Carbs: 22g

Fat: 20g

Protein: 14g

Kale Chips

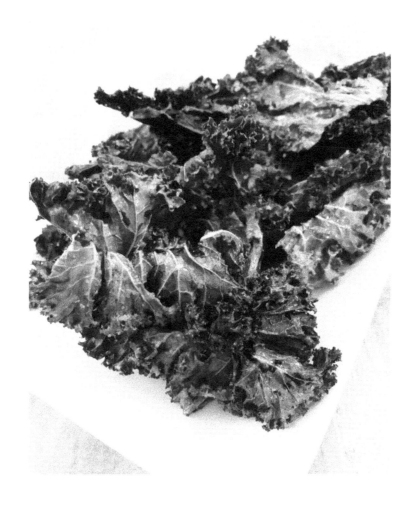

Preparation time: 5 minutes

Cooking time: 25 minutes

Servings: 2

Ingredients:

1 large bunch kale

1 tablespoon extra-virgin olive oil

½ teaspoon chipotle powder

½ teaspoon smoked paprika

¼ teaspoon salt

Directions:

Preheat the oven to 275ºF. Prepare a large baking sheet lined using parchment paper. In a large bowl, stem the kale and tear it into bite-size pieces. Add the olive oil, chipotle powder, smoked paprika, and salt.

Toss the kale with tongs or your hands, coating each piece well. Spread the kale over the parchment paper in a single layer.

Bake within 25 minutes, turning halfway through, until crisp. Cool for 10 to 15 minutes before dividing and storing in 2 airtight containers.

Nutrition:Calories: 100 , Carbs: 9g , Fat: 7g , Protein: 4g

Tempeh-Pimiento Cheese Ball

Preparation time: 5 minutes

Cooking time: 30 minutes

Servings: 8

Ingredients:

8 ounces tempeh, cut into ½ -inch pieces

1 (2-ounce) jar chopped pimientos, drained

¼ cup nutritional yeast

¼ cup vegan mayonnaise, homemade or store-bought

2 tablespoons soy sauce

¾ cup chopped pecans

Directions:

Cook the tempeh within 30 minutes in a medium saucepan of simmering water. Set aside to cool. In a food processor, combine the cooled tempeh, pimientos, nutritional yeast, mayo, and soy sauce. Process until smooth.

Transfer the tempeh mixture to a bowl and refrigerate until firm and chilled for at least 2 hours or overnight.

Toast the pecans in a dry skillet over medium heat until lightly toasted. Set aside to cool.

Shape the tempeh batter into a ball, then roll it in the pecans, pressing the nuts slightly into the tempeh mixture so they stick. Refrigerate within 1 hour before serving.

Nutrition:

Calories: 170

Carbs: 6g

Fat: 14g

Protein: 5g

Peppers and Hummus

Preparation time: 15 minutes

Cooking time: 0 minutes

Servings: 4

Ingredients:

one 15-ounce can chickpeas, drained and rinsed

juice of 1 lemon, or 1 tablespoon prepared lemon juice

¼ cup tahini

3 tablespoons extra-virgin olive oil

½ teaspoon ground cumin

1 tablespoon water

¼ teaspoon paprika

1 red bell pepper, sliced

1 green bell pepper, sliced

1 orange bell pepper, sliced

Directions:

Combine chickpeas, lemon juice, tahini, 2 tablespoons of the olive oil, the cumin, and water in a food processor.

Process on high speed until blended for about 30 seconds. Scoop the hummus into a bowl and drizzle with the remaining tablespoon of olive oil. Sprinkle with paprika and serve with sliced bell peppers.

Nutrition:

Calories: 170

Carbs: 13g

Fat: 12g

Protein: 4g

Drinks

Cookie Dough Milkshake

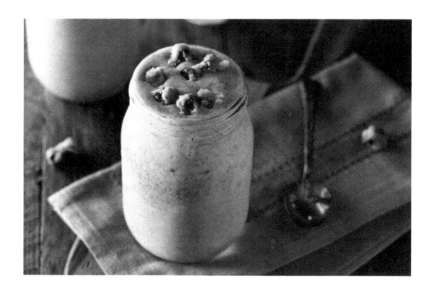

Preparation Time: 5 minutes

Cooking Time: 0 minute

Servings: 2

Ingredients:

2 tablespoons cookie dough

5 dates, pitted

2 teaspoons chocolate chips

1/2 teaspoon vanilla extract, unsweetened

1/2 cup almond milk, unsweetened

1 ½ cup almond milk ice cubes

Directions:

Place all the ingredients in the order in a food processor or blender and then pulse for 2 to 3 minutes at high speed until smooth.

Pour the milkshake into two glasses and then serve with some cookie dough balls.

Nutrition: Calories: 240 Fat: 13g Protein: 21g Sugar: 9g

Strawberry and Hemp Smoothie

Preparation Time: 5 minutes

Cooking Time: 0 minute

Servings: 2

Ingredients:

3 cups fresh strawberries

2 tablespoons hemp seeds

1/2 teaspoon vanilla extract, unsweetened

1/8 teaspoon sea salt

2 tablespoons maple syrup

1 cup vegan yogurt

1 cup almond milk, unsweetened

1 cup of ice cubes

2 tablespoons hemp protein

Directions:

Place all the ingredients in the order in a food processor or blender, except for protein powder, and then pulse for 2 to 3 minutes at high speed until smooth.

Pour the smoothie into two glasses and then serve.

Nutrition: Calories: 510 Fat: 18g Protein: 26g Sugar: 12g

Blueberry, Hazelnut and Hemp Smoothie

Preparation Time: 5 minutes

Cooking Time: 0 minute

Servings: 2

Ingredients:

2 tablespoons hemp seeds

1 ½ cups frozen blueberries

2 tablespoons chocolate protein powder

1/2 teaspoon vanilla extract, unsweetened

2 tablespoons chocolate hazelnut butter

1 small frozen banana

3/4 cup almond milk

Directions:

Place all the ingredients in the order in a food processor or blender and then pulse for 2 to 3 minutes at high speed until smooth.

Pour the smoothie into two glasses and then serve.

Nutrition: Calories: 195 Fat: 14g Protein: 36g Sugar: 10g

Mango Lassi

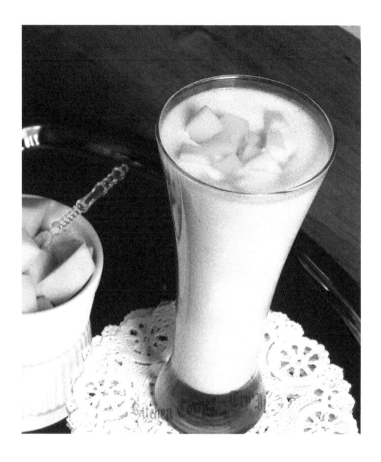

Preparation Time: 5 minutes

Cooking Time: 0 minute

Servings: 2

Ingredients:

1 ¼ cup mango pulp

1 tablespoon coconut sugar

1/8 teaspoon salt

1/2 teaspoon lemon juice

1/4 cup almond milk, unsweetened

1/4 cup chilled water

1 cup cashew yogurt

Directions:

Place all the ingredients in the order in a food processor or blender and then pulse for 2 to 3 minutes at high speed until smooth.

Pour the lassi into two glasses and then serve.

Nutrition: Calories: 420 Fat: 12g Protein: 23g Sugar: 13g

Dessert Recipes

Salted Coconut-Almond Fudge

Preparation Time: 5 minutes

Cooking Time: 0 minutes

Servings: 12

Ingredients:

¾ cup creamy almond butter

½ cup maple syrup

1/3 cup coconut oil, softened or melted

6 tablespoons fair-trade unsweetened cocoa powder

1 teaspoon coarse or flaked sea salt

Directions:

Preparing the Ingredients.

Line a loaf pan with a double layer of plastic wrap. Place one layer horizontally in the pan with a generous amount of overhang. The second layer vertically with a generous amount of overhang.

In a medium bowl, gently mix the almond butter, maple syrup, and coconut oil until well combined and smooth. Add the cocoa powder and gently stir it into the mixture until well combined and creamy.

Pour the mixture into the prepared pan and sprinkle with the sea salt. Bring the overflowing edges of the plastic wrap over the top of the fudge to completely cover it. Place the pan in the freezer for at least 1 hour or overnight, until the fudge is firm.

Remove the pan from the freezer and lift the fudge out of the pan using the plastic-wrap overhangs to pull it out. Transfer to a cutting board and cut into 1-inch pieces.

Nutrition: Calories 297 Fat 20.3 g Carbohydrates 4 g Sugar 5 g Protein 21 g Cholesterol 80 mg

Caramelized Bananas

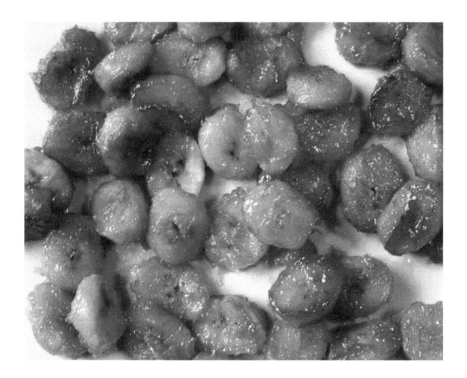

Preparation Time: 5 minutes

Cooking Time: 10 minutes

Servings: 2

Ingredients:

2 tablespoons vegan margarine or coconut oil

2 bananas, peeled, halved crosswise and then lengthwise

2 tablespoons dark brown sugar, demerara sugar, or coconut sugar

2 tablespoons spiced apple cider

Chopped walnuts, for topping

Directions:

Preparing the Ingredients.

Melt the margarine in a nonstick skillet over medium heat. Add the bananas, and cook for 2 minutes. Flip, and cook for 2 minutes more.

Sprinkle the sugar and cider into the oil around the bananas, and cook for 2 to 3 minutes, until the sauce thickens and caramelizes around the bananas. Carefully scoop the bananas into small bowls, and drizzle with any remaining liquid in the skillet. Sprinkle with walnuts.

Nutrition: Calories: 413 Fat: 13g Saturated fat: 4g Cholesterol: 98mg Sodium: 432mg Carbohydrates: 64g Fiber: 5g Protein: 37g

Mixed Berries and Cream

Preparation Time: 10 minutes

Cooking Time: 0 minutes

Servings: 4

Ingredients:

two 15-ounce cans full-fat coconut milk

3 tablespoons agave

½ teaspoon vanilla extract

1-pint fresh blueberries

1-pint fresh raspberries

1-pint fresh strawberries, sliced

Directions:

Preparing the Ingredients.

Refrigerate the coconut milk overnight. When you open the can, the liquid will have separated from the solids. Spoon out the solids and reserve the liquid for another purpose.

In a medium bowl, whisk the agave and vanilla extract into the coconut solids. Divide the berries among four bowls. Top with the coconut cream. Serve immediately.

Nutrition: Calories: 468 Total fat: 19g Saturated fat: 9g Cholesterol: 51mg Sodium: 1041mg Carbohydrates: 53g Fiber: 8g Protein: 23g

"Rugged" Coconut Balls

Preparation Time: 15 minutes

Cooking Time: 0 minute

Servings: 8

Ingredients:

1/3 cup coconut oil melted

1/3 cup coconut butter softened

2 oz coconut, finely shredded, unsweetened

4 Tbsp coconut palm sugar

1/2 cup shredded coconut

Directions:

Combine all ingredients in a blender.

Blend until soft and well combined.

Form small balls from the mixture and roll in shredded coconut.

Place on a sheet lined with parchment paper and refrigerate overnight.

Keep coconut balls into sealed container in fridge up to one week.

Nutrition: Calories: 247 Total Fat: 7g Saturated Fat: 2g Cholesterol: 17mg Sodium: 563mg Carbohydrates: 33g Fiber: 3g Protein: 12g

Conclusion

Congratulations on making it to the end of this cookbook. In numerous surveys, increased admissions of soil-grown foods have been emphatically linked to a decrease in psychological decay. In addition to these, the plant-based diet provides sufficient proteins needed by the body, helps prevent and cure certain diseases and ensures easy weight loss without going hungry. Therefore, following this diet is not only useful for the body but also for the mind, it is a complete diet that does not need any integration and I really hope that this diet is simple and fun for you to replicate.

Good luck!

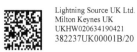

9 781802 523768